Holistic Healing

Your Guide to a Healthier You!

Holistic Healing

Healthy Body Books

http://www.healthybodybooks.com

ISBN-13:
978-1502564399

ISBN-10:
1502564394

The author of this book does not dispense medical advice or prescribe the use of any technique as a form of treatment for physical, emotional, or medical problems without the advice of a physician, either directly or indirectly. The intent of the author is only to offer information of a general nature to help you in your quest for emotional, spiritual and physical well-being. In the event you use any of the information in this book for yourself, which is your constitutional right, the author and the publisher assume no responsibility for your actions. Under no circumstances will any legal responsibility or blame be held against the publisher for any reparation, damages, or monetary loss due to the information herein, either directly or indirectly.

The information herein is offered for informational purposes solely, and is universal as so. The presentation of the information is without contract or any type of guarantee assurance.

The trademarks that are used are without any consent, and the publication of the trademark is without permission or backing by the trademark owner. All trademarks and brands within this book are for clarifying purposes only and are the owned by the owners themselves, not affiliated with this document.

Table Of Contents

Introduction

Have you ever:

-Wondered what Holistic Healing is?

-Tried every western medicine has to offer?

-Are you dissatisfied with Western Medicine?

-Or do you just feel like there must be another way.....

In this book you will discover the most up-to-date information on Alternative Therapies including:

-What is Holistic Healing?

-Benefits of Holistic Healing

-Different types of Holistic Healing such as Aromatherapy and Acupuncture

-The role diet and exercise play in Holistic Healing

- And much more!

Thank you for buying this book, "Holistic Healing: The Ultimate Guide to a Healthier you Today with Holistic Healing!"

A person's wellbeing does not only depend on his physical body. In order to attain a balanced health, people also need to make sure that their emotional, mental and spiritual health is balanced. Holistic Healing has been regarded as the process of restoring balance in the body through different methods.

Holistic healing is different from conventional healing done by other medical professionals. In holistic healing, even non-physical factors are taken into consideration. Practitioners acknowledge that the root cause of most illness is non-physical. Holistic healing is an effective method in achieving overall health and happiness.

I would also like to introduce myself; my name is Simone, the creator of the Healthy Body Books. My deep-seated passion for health has driven me to create these books. Something inside of me has always called out, encouraging me to write books that health-minded individuals would want to read. Health has always been a priority in my life, even when a recent change in my routine made it much more difficult to find myself.

In spite of not feeling my best (or even much like myself), I found ways to continue achieving my goals. After searching long and hard, I found that natural therapies, diets and self-help were enough to help me get things back under control. I found out that these natural remedies were doing so much for me – and I never looked back.

If you are trying to find another way to stay healthy, the Healthy Body Books are for you. If you are anything like me, you might need to find an alternative method to reach your peak. Written by experts in terms that anybody can read, these books are designed to help you identify which aspects of your life just do not seem to be working for you. You should not let anything stop you from being the person you want to be – or from living the life you want to live. This book will help you along you journey.

Good luck!

Keep Up to Date with New Releases

Thank you again for getting yourself a copy of this Book *Holistic Healing: Your Guide to a Healthier You!*

I'd like to offer you the chance to stay up-to date on new books with free access to my newsletter!

You will be getting up to date information on health, fitness and diet, and also get access to getting other Love Your Life for free. By joining my newsletter you will be taking a big step forward in being your Healthiest Body yet!

Just visit http://loveyourlifeseries.comand get free instant access to the Healthy Body Books newsletter today!

Chapter 1: What is Holistic Healing?

When people feel physical pain and discomfort, it is only natural to seek relief through various treatments. **Holistic healing** uses holistic approach in treating ailments. What differentiates it primarily from other medical practices is that it does not necessarily deal with the physical aspect alone.

It is also important to remember that holistic healing cannot be used to replace conventional medical care, but positive results can be attained if this approach is used along with medications prescribed by real medical practitioners. Holistic medication deals with the whole person including his body, mind, emotion and spirit.

The primary goal of holistic healing is to help people find a proper balance in life. Practitioners believe that the human body is composed of interdependent parts where one aspect can affect the other. In order to achieve optimal wellbeing, a person also has to consider the non-physical aspect of his health.

Principles

Holistic healing says that a person needs unconditional love and support in order to be cured.

Holistic healing practitioners believe that people are responsible for their own actions and well-being.

Treatment involves curing the condition and not just alleviating the pain.

Holistic healing highlights the fact that the patient is a person and not a disease.

Everyone has an innate ability to do holistic healing.

8

Role of a Holistic Healer

Holistic healers believe that pain and discomfort are merely symptoms of an inner imbalance. Physical imbalance can be caused by physical exhaustion, lack of exercise and little sleep. People can also suffer from emotional, spiritual and mental imbalance. The role of a holistic healer is to make an evaluation about a person's wellbeing and suggest certain treatments that can help them deal with their problems. Healer can specialize in a specific area of practice.

Holistic Check-up

People who are suffering from any ailment may find comfort in holistic healing. You can evaluate your well being through a basic holistic checkup. A holistic checkup is different from what medical professionals conduct. It usually involves evaluating all aspects of the body.

Where to Find a Holistic Healer?

Holistic healers may include medical professional and homeopathic doctors. You can search the internet for licensed holistic healing practitioners. Here are some tips in choosing a holistic healer.

Get recommendations from people you know. Acupuncture specialists do not provide the same services. Make sure that you ask enough questions from your holistic healing provider.

Research. Try to find as much information about the practitioner as possible. Learn about their training and experience, as well as their specialty.

Your comfort is an important factor in choosing a holistic healer. You should be confident about their skills and trust them enough. Remember that holistic healing involves not only the healer but the patient, as well.

Choose a health care provider who can spend enough time with you. A general check-up can last from 10 to 15 minutes.

Do not be afraid to answer questions. The holistic healing practitioner will need to learn about the person and not just the disease. Additional questions may include emotional balance, exercise, sleeping habits and diet.

Chapter 2: Chakra Alignment

Chakra means wheel in Sanskrit. It defines the wheel of energy that continues to flow in the body. Chakras are considered to be a person's energy centers where life force flows through. Once these chakras are blocked, the body experiences undesirable symptoms. People tend to deal with problems by harnessing emotions that can interfere with the natural flow of energy in the body. Holistic healing aims to align the chakra to balance a person's health.

The Seven Chakras

Root

Root chakra is the first chakra and is called as Muladhara in Sanskrit. It is located at the base of the spine. This chakra is associated with safety and security. It is also known to be the center of manifestation where people take the energy to succeed. If this area is blocked, then a person may become fearful and anxious. The root chakra affects the hips, legs and male sexual energy. The colors of root chakra are red, brown and black.

Holistic healing exercise: Strengthen your root chakra by stomping your feet or by doing squats.

Belly/Sacral

The second chakra is located below the navel and is rooted in the spine. It affects sexuality, self-worth and intuition. This chakra deals with emotions and creativity. Once this chakra is blocked, a person may feel manipulative and obsessed with sex. Physical symptoms include muscle spasm, stiff back and kidney weakness.

The main color associated with the sacral chakra is orange.

Holistic healing exercise: The best exercise to improve sacral energy is pelvis thrust and circular pelvis movements.

Solar Plexus

The third chakra is located two inches below the breastbone and in the center of the stomach. It is generally associated with personal passion, anger, strength and ego. It is also the center of psychic development. Imbalance in the third chakra can result to lack of confidence and confusion. Physical symptoms of imbalance can include food allergies and digestive problems. This chakra is identified with the color yellow.

Holistic healing exercise: Dancing like hoopla hooping and belly dancing can improve your solar plexus energy.

Heart

The fourth chakra is located between the shoulder blades in the back. It regulates love, spirituality and compassion. It directs a person's ability to give and receive love. This chakra also connects the body and mind. Heartaches can cause aura obstructions that can trigger physical symptoms like insomnia, heart attack and high blood pressure. The main colors of the fourth chakra are pink and green.

Holistic healing exercise: Do push-ups and breaststrokes to strengthen your heart chakra.

Throat

Throat is the fifth chakra and is located from the collarbone to the lower back. It is considered as the center of communication, expression, writing and speech. Transformation and healing are also located in this chakra. People with blocked throat chakras can feel weak and timid. The main color for this chakra is light blue.

Holistic healing exercise: Try gargling salt water or singing to improve your throat chakra.

Third Eye

The sixth chakra is situated in the middle of the forehead. It regulates higher intuition and psychic abilities. Imbalance in this chakra can cause headaches and blurred vision. The chakra is associated with dark purple.

Holistic healing exercise: Lucid dreaming and visualization can help you intensify your third eye.

Crown

The crown is the last chakra and is found on the top of the skull. It is the center of spirituality and enlightenment. It is also associated with the flow of wisdom and cosmic awareness. Lack of balance in the crown chakra can lead to depression and frustration. Its main color is white and purple.

Holistic healing exercise: Improve your crown chakra through prayer and meditation.

Holistic Healing and Strengthening your Chakra

Cleaning your chakra is essential in releasing negative vibes and energies.

Comb your aura by using your clean fingers and combing it through your body from the head to the toes. You can wash your hands with running water.

Take a shower. Let the water flow throughout your body. As the water cascades down your body, imagine your troubles and problems flowing along with the water.

Smudge your aura. You can clean your aura by breathing in the smoke of sage, sweet grass, or lavender.

Saltwater soak. Soak your body in warm water with Epsom salt.

Whisk aura with feathers. Use a whisking motion to sweep negative energy surrounding your body. Turkey or owl feather is best used for this cleansing ritual.

Get some sun exposure. Sunshine is essential in the development of the crown chakra, which regulates energy flow.

Stay in a warm room. Your chakras flow better when your body is heated. Having cold hands and feet can prevent energy flow.

Avoid strong breeze. A strong breeze can dull the sensation that you might feel.

Play music as you practice. Listen to instrumental music as you mediate. Let the music flow through you. You might even notice that your chakra energy tends to flow with the music.

Use an elixir. Crystals and gemstones are great tools in increasing your chakra energy. Rub the crystals into your palms to generate chakra flow.

Be patient. Energy flows at a slow rate. It might take you some time before you feel it working.

Uncross your legs. Crossing your legs can prevent the natural flow of energy in your body.

Chapter 3: Breathing and Stress Relief

One of the common mistakes people do is withholding their breath. It is essential to train yourself to breath properly. Proper breathing is needed in maintaining a healthy body.

The Ancient Wisdom of Breathing

People may survive for some time without any food and water, but the human body can only withstand a couple of minutes without breathing. Breathing does not only affect the physical body, but also the mental and spiritual aspect of a person.

Different cultures that explored the secrets of breathing have paved the way for some of the well known holistic healing methods like acupuncture. After the body completes a breathing cycle, an immediate sense of relaxation can be experienced.

Conscious Deep Breathing

Holistic healing employs deep breathing as one of the ways to calm the mind and body. People have to be aware of their breathing pattern.

Soften the belly. Make sure that your diaphragm is relaxed enough to allow your abdomen to rise and fall as you breathe.

Diagnose imbalance. The length of inhalation and exhalation should be ideally the same. If your belly is not moving while you are breathing, then try to relax your abdominal wall.

Stretching. People can encounter breathing difficulties because of tight back muscles. There are many things that can cause sore muscles including stress, lack of physical activity or exhaustion. Stretching and bodywork can also be regarded as holistic healing since these release tension in your muscles and allow you to breathe properly.

Practice breath awareness. Set specific time to practice your breathing. You can practice conscious deep breathing techniques whenever you are in a stressful situation.

Methods of Relieving Stress

Knowing different holistic healing breathing techniques is essential in making sure that you are properly balanced all the time.

Breathing Meditation

Breathing meditation is focused on deep breathing to relax the mind and body. One of its holistic healing advantages is that it can be practiced almost anywhere. The key is to breath from the abdomen. Inhale as much fresh air as possible. The more oxygen you inhale, the less anxious you feel.

Sit comfortably and place one hand in your chest. Breathe through your nose. Observe and make sure that the hand on your stomach will rise and fall with your breathing. Exhale through the mouth while contracting the abdominal muscle. If you find it difficult to breath in a sitting position, then you can also try lying in the floor.

Progressive Muscle Relaxation

Progressive muscle relaxation is a holistic healing approach that has two processes where you tense and relax your muscles. People with muscle spasms should avoid doing this relaxation technique since it can aggravate symptoms. Continuous practice will enable a person to be familiar with the feeling of muscle tension and relaxation.

Start by loosening your clothes and getting into a comfortable position. Take deep breaths to relax your mind. Focus on one body part at a time starting with the right foot. Slowly tense the muscles on your foot and squeeze tightly as you can. Relax your foot and feel the tension flowing away. Shift your attention into another body part and repeat the process. Make sure to take your time and remember to breathe slowly. Remember to focus only on the muscle groups that you want to relax.

Holistic Healing Body-scan Meditation

Body scan meditation is similar to progressive muscle tension but instead of tensing the muscles, it only focuses on the sensation felt on each part of the body.

Lie on your back with your arms stretched to the side. Focus on your breathing and allow yourself to relax. Focus on the toes of your feet and notice any sensation that you might feel. Imagine each breath flowing to your toes. Move your focus to the other parts of your body. Spend extra time on the body parts where you feel pain and discomfort. After completing the process, take time to relax in stillness.

Holistic Healing Mindfulness

Holistic healing mindfulness is the ability to raise awareness regarding your emotions and experiences. A person's self-image can have a negative effect on his physical body. Negative emotions contribute to stress and anxiety. By remaining calm and focused, you can bring back balance into your life. The main purpose of holistic healing and mindfulness meditation is to

18

cultivate a calm mind that can reduce the effects of stress.

Choose a quite place in your house to conduct your meditation. Get into a comfortable position but you should not lie down to avoid falling asleep. Choose a point of focus that can be internal or external. Internal focus can be an imaginary scene and an external focus can be an object. Free your mind from any distracting thoughts. Do not try to fight thoughts that enter your mind, but gently turn your attention back to your point of focus.

Holistic Healing Visualization Meditation

Holistic healing visualization is also referred to as guided imagery where you will be compelled to use all of your senses. This holistic healing technique involves imagining peaceful scenery where you can let go of all anxiety and problems.

Find a quite place to mediate. Close your eyes and remove all your worries. Choose sceneries that can instantly produce calming effects on you. This can be your childhood home or a tropical beach. Picture the scenery as vividly as possible. Include as many sensory details as possible. For example, if you are using the image of a beach for visualization, then try to feel the sand in your feet when you walk or taste the salt in the wind. Welcome the deep relaxation that envelops you. When you are done, slowly open your eyes and return to reality.

Additional Tips

The best way to ensure that these holistic healing techniques will work is by incorporating them into your daily routine. Here are some tips in fitting relaxation techniques in your busy schedule.

Schedule a specific time to meditate each day. Make enough time for two holistic healing meditations. It is easier to meditate in the morning before you start your day.

Practice holistic healing relaxation techniques even in the middle of doing other things. You can meditate on the bus or while waiting for your next appointment.

Include holistic healing techniques in your exercise regimen. Pay attention on how your body is moving as it exercises.

Do not give up. Do not feel discouraged if you skip a few days for meditation. Just resume your practice and slowly build your momentum.

Chapter 4: Auras

People's auras are like magnets that absorb energy. You need to make sure that your aura is constantly balanced to ensure a healthy life. Holistic healing enables a person to be more aware of their auras and how to protect them.

Be Wary of Psychic Vampires

A psychic attack is where a person receives an energy surge from a person who experiences fatigue. People who absorb energies from others are referred to as 'psychic vampires'. This sucking occurs when a person is emotionally unbalanced and he needs to draw energy from other people.

These psychic vampires do not 'suck' energies on purpose. They may not even be aware of what they are doing. However, their actions can negatively affect other people. It is essential for you to understand that anyone can be susceptible to having their energies stolen. The main harm in psychic attack is that there is no exchange of energies and the victim suffers from energy depletion.

A psychic vampire is a person who seeks constant nurturing and guidance. They may also be insecure and want other people's assurance. Symptoms of a psychic attack include loss of energy, dizziness, fatigue and depressed mood.

Protect Yourself from Psychic Vampires

Cross your arms. A person instinctively crosses his arms whenever he wants to protect himself from negative people. When you cross your arms, you instinctively protect your plexus chakra, which is where personal power resides. If you cannot cross your arms, then you can also cross your fingers to prevent psychic vampires from affecting your energy.

Pink. Pink is a calming and nurturing color. Whenever you encounter a negative person, you can close your eyes for a moment and imagine a pink cotton candy. You can also rely on pink gemstones to help you dispel any negative energy.

Improve your immune system. Holistic healing suggests strengthening your immune system to help you combat emotional troubles. When you have a weak body, you are vulnerable to psychic attacks.

Believe. One of the best ways to protect yourself from physic attacks is by believing that the psychic vampire has no right to control your life. You need to take responsibility of your own health and never allow other people to take advantage of you.

Chapter 5: Aromatherapy

Aromatherapy is a popular holistic healing treatment that uses plant scents to heal the body and spirit.

Essential oils

Essential oils are concentrated extracts from plants that were processed through distillation. Essential oils have different effects on the body.

Allspice Berry

This has a warm and spicy scent that is usually associated with masculinity.

Holistic healing benefits: comforting, nurturing and cheering

Amyris

This is also known as West Indian Sandalwood. It has a sweet and woody aroma. It can be blended with other scents like jasmine and cedar wood.

Holistic healing benefits: strengthening

Sweet Basil

Sweet basil has a strong floral and spicy aroma that can last for a long time.

Holistic healing benefits: Uplifting, refreshing and clarifying

Bergamot

Bergamot essential oil comes from the skin of a nearly ripe fruit. It usually smells fruity and sweet. It is used as a deodorizer.

Holistic healing benefits: Inspiring and confidence building

White Camphor

White camphor is associated with cleansing products like soaps and disinfectants.

Holistic healing benefits: Purifying

Cardamom Seed

This oil has floral undertone with a distinctive spicy aroma. It is usually added to masculine scents.

Holistic healing benefits: comforting and alluring

Carrot Seed

The oil extracted from an ordinary carrot can smell sweet and woody. It can be added to other skin care oils.

Holistic healing benefits: Replenishing and restoring

Atlas Cedar

Atlas cedar is found in Algeria and Morocco. Its aroma is associated with oil and animal scent. Atlas essential oil is used in soaps and perfumes.

Holistic healing benefits: Stabilizing and Centering

Red Cedar Wood

Red cedar wood is also known as Juniperus virginiana. It has a balsamic and woody aroma.

Holistic healing benefits: evokes inner strength and combats emotional stress

German Chamomile

German or blue chamomile has a tobacco like scent. It is used in popular soothing oils.

Holistic healing benefits: soothing and relaxing

Cinnamon Leaf

The scent of cinnamon leaf oil is similar to cloves. It is often added in oriental fragrances and skin care products.

Holistic healing benefits: vitalizing and refreshing

Citronella

Citronella has a fresh and woody scent. It is used in household products and outdoor sprays.

Holistic healing benefits: Purifying and vitalizing

Clary Sage

Clary sage has a long lasting bittersweet aroma that can also be mixed with other scents.

Holistic healing benefits: Euphoric and visualizing

Eucalyptus

Eucalyptus has long been used for topical preparations and medicine.

Holistic healing benefits: Invigorating

Frankincense

Frankincense is grown throughout India, Africa and Arabia. This essential oil smells spicy and peppery.

Holistic healing benefits: Visualizing and meditative.

Geranium

Geranium can be found in almost all types of fragrances. It smells like rose with fruity undertone.

Holistic healing benefits: Mood-lifting and balancing.

Lavender

Lavender can be combined with different oils including rosemary, citrus and sage.

Holistic healing benefits: Soothing, balancing and healing

Lemongrass

Lemongrass oil is from a topical grass in Asia. This oil is easily identified by it's lemony and grassy aroma.

Holistic healing benefits: Vitalizing and cleansing

Nutmeg

Nutmeg essential oil is taken from dried nutmegs. It is known for its aromatic and spicy fragrance.

Holistic healing benefits: Rejuvenating and energizing

Peppermint

Peppermint is has a sweet and menthol aroma that can make the sinuses tingle when inhaled.

Holistic healing benefits: Cooling and refreshing

Holistic Healing Ways to Use Essential Oils

You can use essential oil in different ways depending on your needs.

Steam inhalation. Pour two drops of essential oil in a bowl filled with hot water. Place your face near the water and cover your head with clean towel.

Vaporization. Mix five drops of essential oil in a vaporizer. You can also add a few drops in your pillowcase.

Baths. You can add essential oil into your bath water for relaxation and stress relief. Some essential oils can also sooth achy muscles.

Personal care. Add essential oil into your skin care products like lotions and face creams.

Feminine care. Lavender, chamomile and tea tree oil can be used to clean the feminine area.

Compresses. Directly apply the essential oil into the muscle to relieve tension.

Chapter 6: Diet and Exercise

Holistic healing principles include eating the right balance of healthy foods and obtaining proper nutrition. Eating whole, unprocessed foods can prevent many diseases and ailments. Here are some tips in holistic healing diet.

- Try to purchase organic foods when possible.

- Choose foods that contain essential vitamins and nutrients like vegetables, fruits and nuts. Try to choose different colored vegetables. Non-starchy vegetables like carrots, broccoli and beans are also great choices.

- Select whole foods that do not contain any artificial ingredients. Limit your consumption of processed foods.

- Try to eat chicken, turkey and fish at least 2-3 times a week. Remove the skin from the meat before cooking. You can also choose lean pork and sirloin.

- Spices and herbs are great ways to add flavor into your food. As an additional benefit, most herbs have antioxidant benefits.

- Limit sugar intake. Sugar can weaken the immune system and can disrupt the function of the nerves. Since completely eliminating sugar is impossible, try to use natural sweeteners like agave and honey.

- Limit alcohol intake. Alcohol can destroy the neurotransmitters in the brain. It can also negatively affect the gastrointestinal track.

Healthier Comfort Foods

Even the health-conscious people crave for their favorite food sometimes. Fortunately, there are some ways to keep your diet balanced while still enjoying you favorite foods.

Vegetable Mac and Cheese

Mac and cheese is a classic favorite, but it can also contain too many carbohydrates and is high in calories. Try replacing half of your ingredients with mixed vegetables like tomatoes, peas and broccoli.

Pizza

Pizza is one of the most ordered foods in the world. However, most restaurants offer greasy and calorie loaded pizzas. Make your own healthy pizza by choosing whole wheat flour. Top it with a lot of vegetables. Add a strong flavored cheese so that you won't have to add too much salt.

Fried Chicken

Fried chicken can be unhealthy when it is deep fried in oil. You can try cooking your 'fried' chicken in the oven and still retain its delicious flavor. Brown the chickens in the pan and then transfer it in the oven.

Sloppy Joes

Sloppy Joe is a favorite among children and adults. Replace red meat and tomato sauce with turkey meat and whole grain buns. You can also add vegetables in your tomato sauce.

Chicken and Dumplings

Chicken and dumplings have a delectable combination. Make it healthier by choosing chicken breast and adding more vegetables. For the dumpling, make the dough using wheat flour and use herbs for flavoring.

Burgers

Burgers are classic American favorite. You can try a healthier variety by mixing black bean and quinoa to make the patties. Make your own ketchup and add plenty of lettuce and tomato.

Fries

Instead of eating classical potato fries, try sweet potatoes instead. Sweet potatoes contain more nutrients like carotenoids, which is great for eye health.

French Toast

Add cinnamon and fresh fruit into your French toast to make it healthier.

Ice cream Sundae

Ice cream is a delicious dessert and snack. Make it healthier by using pure banana ice cream and topping it with fresh fruit and nuts. You can drizzle chocolate syrup or peanut butter on top for a bit of a treat.

Chocolate Chip Cookies

Add banana, quinoa and dark chocolates into your chocolate chip recipe. Quinoa boosts the protein content and banana provides enough sweetness so you wouldn't have to add much sugar.

Holistic healing exercises

Some people wrongly think that exercise should be physically exhausting for it to be effective. As a result, they engage in difficult workout regimen. Although there is nothing wrong with training hard on your exercise program, it does not have to be painful. Here are four basic **holistic healing** exercises that you can do to improve your body and mind.

Yoga

Most of the yoga forms practiced today have originated in India and Asia. Yoga is considered to be one of the best holistic healing exercises in the world. More and more practitioners are reaping the benefits of this form of exercise. Unlike strenuous workouts, it emphasizes balance and proper breathing. Yoga gives the body a good physical workout while promoting a calm state of mind.

There are many studios that offer holistic healing yoga classes. Beginners should invest in a few classes to make sure that they are doing the proper posture and breathing. Almost anyone can practice yoga. There are easy postures for beginners, but there are also challenging postures for people who have been practicing yoga for a long time.

Qigong

Traditionally, qigong was used to treat ailments and relieve pain. After many years, it became known as one of the few holistic healing exercises that can benefit the body in the long term.

Qigong is a Chinese holistic healing exercise system that highlights physical and mental training. It also combines martial arts and yoga. The movements of the exercise are similar to Eastern martial arts, but it also places great emphasis on holistic healing mindfulness and flexibility. Schools for qigong teach a mix of yoga postures and meditative breathing.

Tai Chi

Tai Chi is a holistic healing method characterized by a slow form of martial art that focuses on physical and mental balance. Its philosophy is based on Taoist and Confucian principles. This ancient art form has been practiced for over half a millennium and is taught in five schools.

Tai Chi is proven effective in curing chronic pain and stress. Unlike yoga and qigong, tai chi is considered to be a legitimate form of martial arts that can be used for protection. Although most holistic healing tai chi classes do not focus much on the martial arts aspect of the exercise, there are still self-defense courses that use tai chi principles.

Massage

Massage can also be categorized as a holistic healing workout since it keeps the body functioning by relaxing tense muscles. It can also improve a person's health by relieving anxiety and stress.

Chapter 7: Acupuncture

Acupuncture is one of the oldest forms of holistic healing. It has originated in China about 2,000 years ago. It became popular in 1971 when a reporter published a story about how the Chinese doctors used needles to relieve his pain.

The term acupuncture defines holistic healing procedures that stimulate specific body parts using needles. Modern holistic healing acupuncture practices derive its techniques from Japan, Korea and China.

Is it safe?

FDA requires licensed holistic healing acupuncture practitioners to use only sterile and safe needles. There are a few complications and problems involved in holistic healing acupuncture practice. Most complications are due to inadequate sterilization process and unskillful use of the needle.

Based on guidelines, holistic healing practitioners should use new and disposable needles for each patient. It is important to remember that when holistic healing acupuncture is not delivered properly, it can cause serious side effects.

Benefits of Acupuncture

Ease Aching Back

Most holistic healing acupuncture patients seek relief from chronic back pain. A clinical study shows that people who tried simulated holistic healing acupuncture treatment where adequate pressure is placed in certain points, but no needle was used experienced better results.

Increases Effectiveness of Medicine

A study in alternative holistic healing medicine revealed that Prozac when combined with acupuncture therapy is as effective at reducing anxiety as a full-dose medicine. Doctors also recommend reducing the dosage and adding holistic healing acupuncture treatments to improve a person's health.

Soothes Indigestion

Holistic healing acupuncture therapy can relieve indigestion and heartburn in pregnant women. Almost 75% of pregnant women who went through acupuncture experienced relief.

Counteracts Radiation Side Effects

Cancer patients who are being treated through radiation experience different side effects. Holistic healing acupuncture can decrease the effect of radiation and relieve symptoms like dry mouth and nausea.

Reduces Persistent Headaches

Holistic healing acupuncture is effective against migraine and headaches. It can also prevent mild symptoms of headache and prevent it from becoming a problem.

Effective for Weight Loss

Holistic healing acupuncture can help people control what they eat. Acupuncture stimulates the release of endorphins that make people feel good. It can also treat digestive problems that cause weight gain.

How to Find a Holistic Healing Licensed Practitioner?

Health care providers can provide you with a detailed list of licensed holistic healing acupuncturists. There is also a national holistic healing acupuncturist organization that can provide suitable referrals.

Make sure to check the holistic healing practitioner's license and credentials. These credentials prove that they have met a certain standard of competency and skill.

Steps to Success Action Plan

"Steps to Success" has been put together to give you somewhere to start on learning about and using Holistic Healing.

To really have success you may need to use this action plan a few times and tried a few different things to get the result you're after. Test, Measure and Monitor need to become your motto until you are feeling happy and healthy!

Step 1- **Assess yourself**. Have you got a health issue that just won't go away, and you don't want to have to take medicine for? Maybe Alternative Therapies can heal you up quickly and easily without taking yucky medicine!

Step 2- **Set REALISTIC expectations**. Everything is trial and error. Just because you try one type of treatment and it doesn't work how you want it to doesn't mean you should give up on Natural Therapies for good. Find the one that works for you, so you can continue going back to it. For me, I always use Chinese Medicine, but I tried a few things before I tried it, now I use it for all my health issues!

Step 3 – **Monitor your Progress**. Keep notes in a diary or journal about your health! It is so handy to be able to look back and now how healthy you were to be able to pick up any changes in your body. Also by doing this you will be able to see if things are taking an affect quicker, or if you need to try a different type of treatment.

Step 4- **Don't Give Up!** Being healthy will be easy to maintain once you know what works for you! Just make sure you take the steps needed to find out what that is!

Step 5 – **Don't be afraid to try new things!** If something isn't working for you change it! Keep changing it until you get it right!

Conclusion

Thank you again for buying this book!

I hope this book was able to help you to fully understand what Holistic Healing is and how it can help you! By being your healthiest self you can offer so much more to yourself and the world.

The next step is to put this knowledge to good use and attempt to get the healthy body you have always dreamed off, you are off to a flying start by reading this book and taking advantage of the Action Plan included.

Finally, if you enjoyed this book, please take the time to share your thoughts and post a review on Amazon. It'd be greatly appreciated!

Thank you and good luck!

http://www.healthybodybooks.com

Other Books You May be Interested In...

Below you'll find some of my other books currently available through Amazon. Healthy Body Books now has over 30 books in the series, so jump on line and check them out today!

Mind, Body, Spirit: The Ultimate Guide to Creating a Strong Mind, Body, Spirit Connection!

The Beginners Guide to Alternative Therapies: The Top 10 Types of Alternative Therapies Explained!

Decided to Detox? 100 Easy Ways to a Healthier You Today

Healthy Living Made Easy: 50 Tips to Living Happy and Healthy!

You can simply search for these amazing titles on the Amazon website.

Free Gift

Thank you again for reading this Book *Holistic Healing: Your Guide to a Healthier You!*

I'd like to reward you with this by offering you free access to my newsletter!

You will be getting up to date information on health, fitness and diet, and also get access to getting other Healthy Body Books for free. By joining my newsletter you will be taking a big step forward in being your Healthiest Body yet!

Just visit http://www.healthybodybooks.com and get free instant access to the Healthy Body Books newsletter today!

Lastly once you finish reading this book would please review this book on Amazon. With your feedback I continue to make this book better and better.

Thank you!

Printed in Great Britain
by Amazon